Ketogenic Diet For Beginners

Quick and Delicious and Low Carb Keto Recipes for Every Meal to Lose Weight, Burn Fat and Transform Your Body

Chloe Roberts

Disclaimer Notice:

Please note the information contained within this document is for educational and entertainment purposes only. All effort has been executed to present accurate, up to date, and reliable, complete information. No warranties of any kind are declared or implied. Readers acknowledge that the author is not engaging in the rendering of legal, financial, medical or professional advice. The content within this book has been derived from various sources. Please consult a licensed professional before attempting any techniques outlined in this book.

By reading this document, the reader agrees that under no circumstances is the author responsible for any losses, direct or indirect, which are incurred as a result of the use of information contained within this document, including, but not limited to, errors, omissions, or inaccuracies.

Table of Content

Introduction

Thank you for purchasing **Ketogenic Diet For Beginners: Quick and Delicious and Low Carb Keto Recipes for Every Meal to Lose Weight, Burn Fat and Transform Your Body**

The ketogenic diet is a dietary regimen that drastically reduces carbohydrates, while increasing proteins and especially fats. The main purpose of this imbalance in the proportions of macronutrients in the diet is to force the body to use fats as a source of energy.

In the presence of carbohydrates, in fact, all cells use their energy to carry out their activities. But if these are reduced to a sufficiently low level they begin to use fats, all except nerve cells that do not have the ability to do so. A process called ketosis is then initiated, because it leads to the formation of molecules called ketone bodies, this time usable by the brain. Typically ketosis is achieved after a couple of days with a daily carbohydrate intake of about 20-50 grams, but these amounts can vary on an individual basis.

BREAKFAST

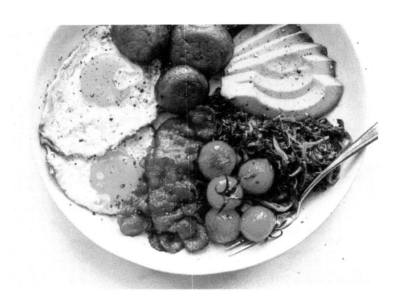

Keto Avocado with Bacon

Preparation Time: 5 minutes

Cooking Time: 20 minutes

Servings: 1

Ingredients:

*   4 hard-boiled egg

*   1 pc avocado

*   2 tbsp. olive oil

*   100 g bacon

*   salt and pepper

Directions:

1.   Preheat oven to 350 ° F.

2.   In a pan that filled of water, put the egg. Set to a boil and let it brew for 8-10 minutes. Place the eggs in ice water immediately after preparation to make them easier to clean.

3.   Cut the eggs in half and dig up the yolks. Place them in a small bowl.

4.   Add avocado, butter, and mashed potatoes until salt and pepper are mixed to taste.

5.   Set the bacon on a baking sheet then bake until crispy. It takes about 5-7 minutes.

6.   Using a spoon, carefully add the mixture back to the cooked egg whites and set the sails with bacon! Enjoy it!

Nutrition: Pure carbohydrates: 1 g Fats: 13 g Proteins: 5 g Calories: 144

Egg Keto Cupcakes

Preparation Time: 10 minutes

Cooking Time: 25 minutes

Servings: 6

Ingredients:

- 2 pcs green onions finely chopped green onions

- 150 g Sausages of sliced sausages or bacon

- 12 pcs Egg

- 2 tbsp. l Pesto

- Salt and pepper

- 175 g grated cheese

Directions:

1. Preheat the oven to 350 ° F.

2. Lubricate the muffin pan with butter.

3. Fill onions and sausages at the bottom of the molds.

4. Beat the eggs with pesto, salt, and pepper. Add cheese and mix thoroughly.

5. Fill the cupcake pan with the resulting mixture.

6. Bake in the oven for 15-20 minutes depending on the size of the mold.

Nutrition: Carbohydrates: 2 g Fats: 26 g P roteins: 23 g Kcal: 336

Cacao Crunch Cereal

Preparation Time: 5 minutes

Cooking Time: 0 minutes

Servings: 2

Ingredients:

- ½ cup slivered almonds

- 2 tablespoons coconut, shredded or flakes

- 2 tablespoons chia seeds

- 2 tablespoons cacao nibs

- 2 tablespoons sunflower seeds

- Unsweetened nondairy milk of choice (I use macadamia milk), for serving

Directions:

1. In a small bowl, mix the almonds, coconut, chia seeds, cacao nibs, and sunflower seeds. Divide between two bowls.

2. Pour in the nondairy milk and serve.

Nutrition: Calories: 325 Total Fat: 27 Protein: 10g Total Carbs: 17g Fiber: 12g Net Carbs: 5g

KETO BREAD

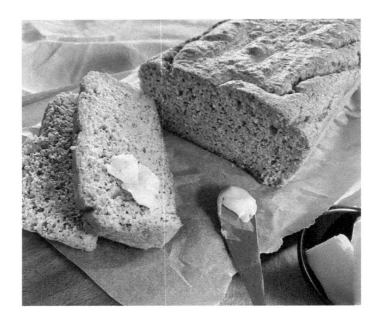

Puri Bread

Preparation Time: 10 minutes

Cooking Time: 5 minutes

Servings: 6

Ingredients:

* 1 cup almond flour, sifted

* 1/2 cup of warm water

* 2 Tbsp. clarified butter

* 1 cup olive oil for frying

* Salt to taste

Directions:

1. Salt the water and add the flour.

2. Build a hole in the center of the dough and pour warm clarified butter.

3. Knead the dough and let stand for 15 minutes, covered.

4. Shape into 6 balls.

5. Flatten the balls into 6 thin rounds using a rolling pin.

6. Heat enough oil to completely cover a round frying pan.

7. Place a puri in it when hot.

8. Fry for 20 seconds on each side.

9.   Place on a paper towel.

10.   Repeat with the rest of the puri and serve.

Nutrition: Calories: 106 Fat: 3g Carb: 5g

Cracked Wheat Bread:

Preparation time: 2 hours

Cooking time: 3 hours

Servings: 8

Ingredients:

- 325 ml warm water
- 1/2 cup (62.5 g) Cracked Wheat Hot Cereal, uncooked
- 2 tablespoons (30 g) pressed light or dim darker sugar
- 14 g margarine or 15 ml vegetable oil, for example, canola
- 125 g Stone Ground Whole Grain Whole Wheat Graham Flour
- 218.8 g Bread Flour
- 9 g salt
- 9 g Fast-Rise Yeast

Directions:

1. Spot ingredients in bread skillet as indicated by maker's bearings. Select the entire wheat cycle and begin the machine.

2.   Yield: 682.5-g portion

3.   Set machine on the mixture cycle. When the cycle is processed, structure batter into a loaf and spot in lubed 22.5 cm x 12.5 cm x 7.5-cm container.

4.   Enable the second ascent to top of container and heat in 350°F stove for about 35 - 40 minutes or until moment read thermometer embedded in focus enrolls at any rate 190°. Turn out onto wire rack to cool.

Nutrition: Cal: 287, Carbs: 1 g Fiber: 10 g, Fat: 11 g, Protein: 26 g, Sugars: 1 g.

Flax Prairie Bread:

Preparation time: 2 hours

Cooking time: 3 hours

Servings: 8

Ingredients:

- 295 ml warm water

- 40 g golden nectar

- 28 ml vegetable oil, for example, canola

- 47 g Milled Flax Seed

- 125 g Stone Ground Whole Grain Whole Wheat Graham Flour

- 250 g Bread Flour

- 9 g salt

- 30 g broiled sunflower seeds, hulled and unsalted

- 1 tablespoon (8 g) poppy seeds

- 8 g Fast-Rise Yeast

Directions:

1. Spot ingredients in bread dish as indicated by producer's headings. Select the entire wheat cycle and begin the machine.

2.   Yield: 682.5-g loaf

3.   Set machine on the mixture cycle. When the cycle is processed, structure batter into a loaf and spot in lubed 22.5 cm x 12.5 cm x 7.5-cm container.

4.   Enable the second ascent to top of container and heat in 350F stove for about 35 - 40 minutes or until moment read thermometer embedded in focus enrolls at any rate 190. Turn out onto wire rack to cool.

Nutrition: Cal: 213, Carbs: 2 g Fiber: 10 g, Fat: 11 g, Protein: 26 g, Sugars: 1 g.

Caraway Rye Bread:

Preparation time: 1 hour

Cooking time: 2 hours

Servings: 4

Ingredients:

- 235 ml warm water

- 40 g nectar

- 40 g molasses

- 14 g spread

- 9 g salt

- 4.2 g caraway seeds

- 0.8 g ground orange get-up-and-go

- 125 g Organic Stone Ground Whole Grain Rye Flour

- 250 g Organic Naturally White Unbleached, All-Purpose Flour

- 14 g Vital Wheat Gluten

- 10 g yeast

Directions:

1. Place all ingredients in the bread dish as indicated by the producer's directions. Select the entire wheat setting and begin the machine.

2. Yield: a 682.5-g loaf

3. Set machine on batter cycle. When the process is finished, structure the mixture into a loaf and spot in lubed 22.5 cm x 12.5 cm x 7.5-cm dish.

4. Enable the second ascent to the top of the plate and prepare in 350F broiler for about 35 -40 minutes or until moment read thermometer embedded in focus enrolls in any event 190F.

Nutrition: Cal: 254, Carbs: 2 g Fiber: 8 g, Fat: 11 g, Protein: 25 g, Sugars: 1 g.

Mocha Java Bread:

Preparation time: 1 hour

Cooking time: 2 hours

Servings: 4

Ingredients:

- 175 ml warm water

- 218.8 g Bread Flour

- 8 g nonfat dry milk

- 6 g salt

- 21 g spread, relaxed

- 31.3 g Stone Ground Whole Grain Rye Flour

- 22.5 g stuffed light or dim dark colored sugar

- One huge egg

- 7.2 g moment mocha espresso blend with sugar

- 40 g hacked walnuts

- 4 g Fast-Rise Yeast

Directions:

1.   Place all ingredients in a bread dish as indicated by the maker's directions. Select the entire cycle and begin the

machine. Yield: One I-pound (455-g) normal or 11/2-pound (682.5-g) huge loaf

2.   Set machine on batter cycle. When the process is finished, structure the mixture into a loaf and spot in lubed 9 x 5 x 3-inch (22.5 x 12.5 x 7.5-cm) container.

3.   Enable the second ascent to the top of the skillet and prepare in 350F broiler for about 35 - 40 minutes or until moment read thermometer embedded in focus enlists in any event 190F. Turn out to wire rack to cool.

Nutrition: Cal: 321, Carbs: 4 g Fiber: 2 g, Fat: 9 g, Protein: 21 g, Sugars: 2 g.

Cracked Wheat Sunflower Bread:

Preparation time: 2 hours

Cooking time: 3 hours

Servings: 8

Ingredients:

• 235 ml warm water

• 1 tablespoon (14 g) spread, diminished or 1 tablespoon (15 ml) vegetable oil,

• 1 tablespoon (20 g) nectar

• 1 tablespoon (8 g) nonfat dry milk

• 6 g salt

• 281.3 g Bread Flour

• 31.3 g Cracked Wheat Hot Cereal, uncooked

• 1/4 cup (35 g) broiled sunflower seeds, hulled and unsalted

• 4 g Fast-Rise Yeast

Directions:

1. Spot ingredients in bread dish as indicated by producer's headings. Select the essential cycle and begin the machine.

2.   Yield: 682.5-g portion

3.   Set machine on the mixture cycle. When the cycle is processed, structure batter into a loaf and spot in lubed 22.5 cm x 12.5 cm x 7.5-cm container.

4.   Enable the second ascent to top of container and heat in 350F stove for about 35 - 40 minutes or until moment read thermometer embedded in focus enrolls at any rate 190. Turn out onto wire rack to cool.

Nutrition: Cal: 287, Carbs: 1 g Fiber: 10 g, Fat: 11 g, Protein: 26 g, Sugars: 1 g.

Whole Wheat Carrot Bread:

Preparation time: 3 hours

Cooking time: 3 hours

Servings: 6

Ingredients:

• 120 ml warm water

• 6 g salt

• 79.2 g ground crisp carrots (around 1 enormous)

• 1 tablespoon (20 g) nectar

• 2 tablespoons (30 g) plain, low-fat yogurt

• 1 tablespoon (20 g) molasses

• 1 tablespoon (13.6 g) vegetable oil

• 16.6 g Bread Flour

• 82.5 g Stone Ground Whole Grain Whole Wheat

Graham Flour

• 2g nonfat dry milk

• 2 tablespoons (18 g) slashed pecans (discretionary)

• 4 g Fast-Rise Yeast

Directions:

1.   Place ingredients in bread dish as per maker's headings. Select the entire wheat cycle and begin the machine.

2.   Yield: 455-g ordinary or 682.5-g huge portion

3.   Set machine on the mixture cycle. When the cycle is processed, structure batter into a loaf and spot in lubed 22.5 cm x 12.5 cm x 7.5-cm container.

4.   Enable the second ascent to top of container and heat in 350F stove for about 35 - 40 minutes or until moment read thermometer embedded in focus enrolls at any rate 190. Turn out onto wire rack to cool.

Nutrition: Cal: 321, Carbs: 2 g Fiber: 12 g, Fat: 13 g, Protein: 35 g, Sugars: 1 g.

Old-Fashioned Rye Bread:

Preparation time: 3 hours

Cooking time: 2 hours

Servings: 5

Ingredients:

• 355 ml warm water

• 45 g stuffed light or dim dark colored sugar

• 12 g salt

• 30 ml of vegetable oil

• 170 g molasses

• 85 g nectar

• 5g ground orange strip

• 312.5 g Organic Stone Ground Whole Grain Rye Flour

• 250 g Organic Naturally White Unbleached All-Purpose Flour

• 20 g Fast-Rise Yeast

Directions:

1. Stone Ground Whole Grain Yellow Corn Meal, Plain, for sprinkling

2.   Spot water, darker sugar, salt, oil, molasses, nectar, orange strip, flours, and yeast in bread container as indicated by maker's bearings. Select the mixture cycle.

3.   When the cycle is finished, move the mixture to a floured surface and shape into two round portions. Spot on marginally lubed treat sheet sprinkled with corn supper. Spread with soggy fabric and let it ascend for around 60 minutes.

4.   Preheat broiler to 375F.

5.   Heat for 35 to 40 minutes or until the moment read thermometer embedded in focus enrolls at any rate 190°F. Move to a wire rack to cool.

6.   Yield: a 682.5-g loaf

Nutrition: Cal: 216, Carbs: 1 g Fiber: 3 g, Fat: 10 g, Protein: 13 g, Sugars: 1 g.

Multi-Grain and More Bread:

Preparation time: 3 hours

Cooking time: 2 hours

Servings: 5

Ingredients:

- 175 ml warm water

- 156.3 g Bread Flour

- 31.3 g Stone Ground Whole Grain Whole Wheat

Graham Flour

- 8 g nonfat dry milk

- 6 g salt

- 7 g Multi-Grain Cereal with Flaxseed, uncooked

- 14 g Wheat Germ, Untoasted

- 30 g nectar

- 4 g Fast-Rise Yeast

Directions:

1. Place all ingredients in the bread dish as per the maker's headings. Select the entire cycle and begin the machine.

2. Yield: 455-g normal or 682.5-g huge loaf

3.   Set machine on batter cycle. When a process is finished, structure the batter into a loaf and spot it in a lubed 22.5 cm x 12.5 cm x 7.5 cm container.

4.   Enable the second ascent to the top of the skillet and prepare in 350F stove for about 35 - 40 minutes or until a moment read thermometer embedded in focus enlists at any rate 190F.

5.   Turn out onto wire rack to cool.

Nutrition: Cal: 267, Carbs: 3 g Fiber: 4 g, Fat: 12 g, Protein: 23 g, Sugars: 2 g.

Low-Carb Garlic & Herb Focaccia Bread

Preparation Time: 10 minutes

Cooking Time: 25 min

Serving: 7

Ingredients:

- 1 cup Almond Flour

- 1/4 cup Coconut Flour

- 1/2 teaspoon Xanthan Gum

- 1 teaspoon Garlic Powder

- 1 teaspoon Flaky Salt

- 1/2 teaspoon heating Soda

- 1/2 teaspoon heating Powder

- Wet Ingredients

- 2 eggs

- 1 teaspoon Lemon Juice

- 2 teaspoon Olive oil + 2 teaspoons of Olive Oil to sprinkle

- Top with Italian Seasoning and TONS of flaky salt!

Directions:

1.   Heat broiler to 350 and line a preparing plate or 8-inch round dish with the material.

2.   Whisk together the dry fixings ensuring there are no knots.

3.   Beat the egg, lemon squeeze, and oil until joined.

4.   Merge the wet and the dry together, working rapidly, and scoop the mixture into your dish.

5.   Make sure not to blend the wet and dry until you are prepared to place the bread in the broiler on the grounds that the raising response starts once it is blended!!!

6.   Bake secured for around 10 minutes. Sprinkle with Olive Oil heat for an extra 10-15 minutes revealing to dark-colored tenderly.

7.   Top with increasingly flaky salt, olive oil (discretionary), a scramble of Italian flavoring and crisp basil. Let cool totally before cutting for an ideal surface!!

Nutrition: Cal: 80, Carbs: 1g Fiber: 8.5 g, Fat: 7 g, Protein: 8g, Sugars: 10 g.

Cauliflower Bread with Garlic & Herbs

Preparation Time: 9 minutes

Cooking Time: 26 min

Serving: 12

Ingredients:

• 3 cup Cauliflower ("riced" utilizing nourishment processor*)

• 10 enormous Egg (isolated)

• 1/4 teaspoon Cream of tartar (discretionary)

• 1 1/4 cup Coconut flour

• 1 1/2 teaspoon sans gluten heating powder

• 1 teaspoon Sea salt

• 6 teaspoon Butter (unsalted, estimated strong, at that point softened; can utilize ghee for sans dairy)

• 6 cloves Garlic (minced)

• 1 teaspoon Fresh rosemary (slashed)

• 1 teaspoon Fresh parsley (slashed)

Direction:

1. Preheat the broiler to 350 degrees F (177 degrees C). Line a 9x5 in (23x13 cm) portion skillet with material paper.

2.   Steam the riced cauliflower. You can do this in the microwave (cooked for 3-4 minutes, shrouded in plastic) OR in a steamer bin over water on the stove (line with cheesecloth if the openings in the steamer container are too huge, and steam for a couple of moments). The two different ways, steam until the cauliflower is delicate and delicate. Enable the cauliflower to sufficiently cool to deal with.

3.   Meanwhile, utilize a hand blender to beat the egg whites and cream of tartar until solid pinnacles structure.

4.   Place the coconut flour, preparing powder, ocean salt, egg yolks, dissolved margarine, garlic, and 1/4 of the whipped egg whites in a nourishment processor.

5.   When the cauliflower has cooled enough to deal with, envelop it by kitchen towel and press a few times to discharge however much dampness as could reasonably be expected. (This is significant - the final product ought to be dry and bunch together.) Add the cauliflower to the nourishment processor. Procedure until all-around joined. (Blend will be thick and somewhat brittle.)

6. Add the rest of the egg whites to the nourishment processor. Overlay in only a bit, to make it simpler to process. Heartbeat a couple of times until simply consolidated. (Blend will be cushioned.) Fold in the hacked parsley and rosemary. (Don't over-blend to abstain from separating the egg whites excessively.)

7. Transfer the player into the lined heating skillet. Smooth the top and adjust somewhat. Whenever wanted, you can squeeze more herbs into the top (discretionary).

Nutrition: Cal: 70, Carbs: 2.5 g, Fiber: 4.5 g, Fat: 15 g, Protein: 4g, Sugars: 3 g.

Grain-Free Tortillas Bread

Preparation Time: 5 minutes

Cooking Time: 20 min

Serving: 5

Ingredients:

- 96 g almond flour
- 24 g coconut flour
- 2 teaspoons thickener
- 1 teaspoon heating powder
- 1/4 teaspoon fit salt
- 2 teaspoons apple juice vinegar
- 1 egg softly beaten
- 3 teaspoons water

Directions:

1. Add almond flour, coconut flour, thickener, preparing powder and salt to nourishment processor. Heartbeat until completely joined. Note: you can, on the other hand, whisk

everything in a huge bowl and utilize a hand or stand blender for the accompanying advances.

2.	Pour in apple juice vinegar with the nourishment processor running. When it has dispersed equally, pour in the egg. Pursued by the water, stop the nourishment processor once the batter structures into a ball. The batter will be clingy to contact.

3.	Wrap mixture in stick film and ply it through the plastic for a moment or two. Consider it somewhat like a pressure ball. Enable the mixture to rest for 10 minutes (and as long as three days in the refrigerator).

4.	Heat up a skillet (ideally) or container over medium warmth. You can test the warmth by sprinkling a couple of water beads if the drops vanish promptly your dish are excessively hot. The beads should 'go' through the skillet.

5.	Break the mixture into eight 1" balls (26g each). Turn out between two sheets of material or waxed paper with a moving pin or utilizing a tortilla press (simpler!) until each round is 5-crawls in distance across.

6.   Transfer to skillet and cook over medium warmth for only 3-6 seconds (significant). Flip it over promptly (utilizing a meager spatula or blade), and keep on cooking until just daintily brilliant on each side (however with the customary roasted imprints), 30 to 40 seconds. The key isn't to overcook them, as they will never again be flexible or puff up.

7.   Keep them warm enclosed by kitchen fabric until serving. To rewarm, heat quickly on the two sides, until simply warm (not exactly a moment)

Nutrition: Cal: 70, Carbs: 2.2g Fiber: 4.5 g, Fat: 8 g, Protein: 8g, Sugars: 3 g.

KETO PASTA

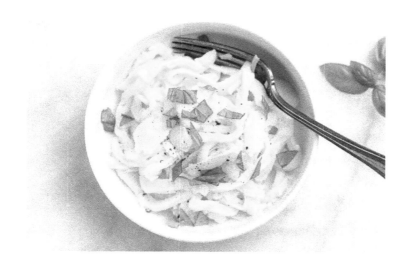

Lemon Chicken with Angel Hair Pasta

Preparation time: 10 minutes

Cooking time: 25 minutes

Servings: 3

Ingredients

- Shirataki angel hair noodles (2–7-ounce packages)

- Chicken breast (1 pound)

- XCT Oil/another cooking oil (1 tablespoon)

- Organic garlic (1 large clove)

- Dried oregano (.5 teaspoon) or Minced fresh oregano–leaves only (1 teaspoon)

- Himalayan pink salt (.5 teaspoon)

- Large lemon (1)

- Butter or ghee (2 tablespoons)

- Collagelatin/another grass-fed gelatin (1 tablespoon)

- For the Garnish: Fresh oregano–leaves only (1-2 tablespoons)

Directions:

1. Rinse the noodles. Drain the noodles and arrange them in a dry skillet using the medium temperature heat setting.

"Dry roast" them for 1 minute). Cool in the pan for 2-3 minutes.

2.   In the meantime, warm a large cast-iron skillet using the med-high temperature setting. Pour in the oil.

3.   Dice the chicken into small chunks and toss into the skillet with the minced garlic, salt, and dried oregano.

4.   Sauté until fully cooked (8-10 minutes). Stir occasionally. Transfer the chicken into a mixing bowl. Set aside.

5.   Reduce the skillet temperature setting to medium. Next, add butter and stir until melted. Whisk in the Collagelatin to finish.

6.   Fold the noodles and chicken back into the skillet, tossing to combine.

7.   Serve topped with lemon zest and a garnish of fresh oregano.

Nutrition: Calories: 398 Fat: 21 g Carb: 4 g Protein: 28 g

Fresh Egg Pasta

Preparation time: 10 minutes

Cooking time: 35 minutes

Servings: 4

Ingredients

*   Coconut flour (3 tablespoons)

*   Almond flour (1 cup)

*   Kosher salt (.25 teaspoon)

*   Xanthan gum (2 teaspoons)

*   Apple cider vinegar (2 teaspoons)

*   Egg (1)

*   Water (2-4 teaspoons–as needed)

*   Olive oil (2 tablespoons)

*   Grass-fed unsalted butter (.25 cup or as needed)

*   Optional: Garlic cloves–slivered (4)

Directions:

1.   Measure and sift the almond flour, coconut flour, xanthan gum, and salt into a food processor. Pulse until thoroughly combined.

2.   Pour in the vinegar with the food processor running. Add in the egg. Add water by the teaspoon, as needed, until the dough forms into a ball. The dough should be firm, yet sticky to the touch and with no creases (if the dough is dry, add a little more water).

3.   Merge dry ingredients to a large bowl and whisk until thoroughly combined. Pour in the vinegar and whisk well. Pour in the egg while whisking vigorously until the dough becomes too stiff to whisk. Knead the dough until thoroughly incorporated—adding a teaspoon of water at a time as needed.

4.   For farfalle (bows): Roll out the pasta to its thinnest point using a tortilla press between parchment paper or a pasta machine. You can also use a rolling pin, but it'll take a little longer. Cut into 2 by 1-inch rectangles.

5.   Place the shaped pasta in the freezer for at least 15 minutes.

6.   Dissolve the butter in a skillet and attach the garlic. When the garlic begins to brown, fold in the chilled pasta, and baste right away.

7.   Cook the pasta until it just begins to get some color for an 'al dente' texture (soft with a bite). Serve right away with toppings of choice.

Nutrition: Calories: 143 Fat: 23 g Carb: 3 g Protein: 15 g

Chicken and Pasta Soup

Preparation time: 5 minutes

Cooking Time: 30 minutes

Serving Size: 6

Ingredients:

- 1 sprig fresh thyme

- 5 cups chicken broth

- 1 cup (orzo shaped) pasta

- 3 cups cooked chicken

- 1 bay leaf

- 1 tablespoon olive oil

- 1 rib celery (minced)

- 1/2 teaspoon kosher salt

- 1 carrot (shredded)

- 1/2 medium onion (diced)

- 1 clove garlic (minced)

Directions:

1. Bring a big pot of ice water over medium temperature to a boil and sprinkle it with salt generously.

2.	Add the pasta and simmer until al dente, stirring regularly, for around ten minutes and drain.

3.	In the meantime, on medium heat, melt the butter in a big saucepan.

4.	Insert the onions, garlic, carrots, celery, and salt; simmer for around ten minutes, until soft.

5.	Transfer the veggies to the poultry, bay leaf, chives, and broth, bring to a simmer for ten minutes.

6.	Just prior to eating, add the pasta to the soup. Serve into warm cups.

7.	Soup can be cooked and frozen in advance, only exclude the pasta and substitute it while serving.

Nutrition: Calories: 231 Fat,: 11 g Carb1 3 g Protein: 13 g

Lemon Garlic Shrimp with Zucchini Pasta

Preparation time: 10 minutes

Cooking time: 25 minutes

Servings: 3

Ingredients

- Medium zucchini (4)

- Raw shrimp (1.5 pounds or about 30)

- Olive oil (2 tablespoons)

- Garlic cloves (4)

- Butter or ghee (2 tablespoons)

- Lemon (1 for juice and zest)

- Chicken broth/White wine (.25 cup)

- Chopped parsley (.25 cup)

- Red pepper flakes (a pinch)

- Black pepper and salt (as desired)

Directions:

1. Rinse and discard the ends from each zucchini and slice the 'pasta' using a spiralizer. Finely dice the garlic cloves. Peel and devein the shrimp.

2.   Warm the olive oil in a skillet using the med-high temperature setting. Toss in the shrimp in a flat layer using a dusting of pepper and salt. Sauté for one minute, but don't stir.

3.   Chop and add the garlic and shrimp. Sauté for another one to two minutes on the second side. Transfer the shrimp into a platter.

4.   Mix in the butter, lemon juice, zest, white wine, and red pepper flakes into the pan. Simmer for two to three minutes.

5.   Sprinkle the parsley and fold in the zucchini pasta. Toss for about 30 seconds to warm it up. Fold in the shrimp and sauté for about one more minute before serving.

Nutrition: Calories: 345 Fat: 25 g Carb: 5 g Protein: 15 g

Vietnamese Pasta Bowl

Preparation time: 20 minutes

Cooking time: 25 minutes

Servings: 1

Ingredients:

- A pinch of salt

- A quarter pounder of shrimp Butterfield

- 25 grams of chopped peanuts

- Half a cup of cucumber

- Four(4) cups of romaine's lettuces (chopped)

- 25 great of pork ribs(thinly cut)

- Two (2) packs of Shirataki noodles (rinsed and drained)

- Nine (9) sprigs of cilantro

- 20 grams of sprouted mung beans

- A pound of boneless country style

- A quarter cup of fish sauce (Red coat)

- Two (2) tablespoons of white rice vinegar

- A quarter cup of water

- Two (2) tablespoons of Erythritol

- A tablespoon spoon of garlic chili sauce

Directions:

1.   Boil the noodles for 3-5 minutes, then drain.

2.   Put the noodles in the fridge until the salad is ready to be served.

3.   Sprinkle some salt on shrimps and pork ribs and grill until well cooked, then set aside.

4.   Share the already prepared sales ingredients into four different bowls.

5.   Note: The bowls should be big enough to stir and toss salad in without spilling.

6.   Put the cooked noodles, romaine, cooked shrimp and pork, cilantro, peanuts, cucumber and mung beans.

7.   Put fish sauce, white rice vinegar, garlic chili sauce, Erythritol and water in a bowl and mix until well combined.

8.   Drizzle a generous amount over your salad, then toss to combine. Serve as desired.

Nutrition: Calories: 300 Total Fat: 17g Carbs: 4g Protein: 31g

Marinara Zoodles

Preparation time: 10 minutes

Cooking time: 25 minutes

Servings: 3

Ingredients

• Olive oil (2 tablespoons)

• Garlic cloves (6)

• White onions (.5 cup)

• Tomatoes (14 ounces)

• Tomato paste (2 tablespoons)

• Basil leaves (.5 cup–loosely packed)

• Freshly cracked black pepper (.25 teaspoon)

• Cayenne (1 pinch)

• Spiralized zucchinis (2 large)

• Coarse salt (1.5 teaspoons)

Directions:

1. Heat the skillet and pour oils into it.

2. Mince the garlic cloves, onions, and tomatoes. Roughly chop the basil leaves. Use a veggie peeler or spiralizer to prepare the zucchini.

3.   Toss in and sauté the onion for about five minutes before adding in the garlic. Sauté the onions for 60 seconds.

4.   Mix in the salt, basil, crushed red pepper flakes, pepper, tomato paste, and tomatoes. Combine thoroughly.

5.   Simmer the sauce and lower the heat to medium-low. Simmer until the oil takes on a deep-orange color, which indicates the sauce is thickened and reduced.

6.   Add in the noodles and let them soften approximately two minutes before serving.

Nutrition: Calories: 345 Fat: 25 g Carb: 5 g Protein: 15 g

Keto Shrimp Scampi

Preparation time: 20 minutes

Cooking time: 10 minutes

Servings: 1

Ingredients:

- A quarter cup of chicken broth

- A quarter teaspoon of red chili flakes

- A pinch of salt

- One pound of shrimp

- A clove of garlic (minced)

- Two (2) tablespoons of parsley (chopped)

- Two (2) tablespoons of lemon juice

- Two (2) tablespoons of unsalted butter

- Two (2) summer squash

Directions:

1. Slice the squash.

2. Sprinkle with salt and spread the noodles on an absorbent piece of parchment or paper towel, set aside for 15 minutes.

3.   Use the paper towel to wring out the excess moisture in the noodles.

4.   In a non-stick pan, melt butter, and stir fry garlic until it starts to turn brown.

5.   Add lemon juice, chicken broth and chili flakes, stir and set on medium-low for 3 minutes.

6.   Merge the shrimp, let boil for another 3 minutes or until shrimps start to turn a light shade of pink, then reduce the heat to low and let it simmer.

7.   Taste the sauce and add pepper and salt to your liking.

8.   Put in the summer squash noodles and parsley, stirring gently so as to coat the noodles in the sauce.

Nutrition: Calories: 334 Total Fat: 13.1g Carbs: 2.49g Protein: 48.4g

Keto Shirataki Noodles

Preparation time: 2 minutes

Cooking time: 3 minutes

Servings: 1

Ingredients:

- A tablespoon of unsalted butter
- A quarter cup of grated Parmesan
- A quarter teaspoon of garlic powder
- A quarter teaspoon of Kosher salt
- A quarter teaspoon of black Pepper
- A pack of miracle noodles

Directions:

1. Drain and rinse noodles because they tend to have a fishy smell.

2. Put a large pan on medium-low and dry-roast the noodles.

3. Add butter, salt, garlic powder, and pepper. Stir fry.

4. Turn off the heat and put the noodles into a plate.

5. Sprinkle some parmesan cheese and serve.

Nutrition: Calories: 0 Total Fat: 0g Carbs: 0g Protein: 0g

Zoodles with Sardines, Capers, and Tomatoes

Preparation time: 10 minutes

Cooking time: 8 minutes

Servings2 3

Ingredients

- Brisling sardines packed in olive oil (4-ounce can)

- Olive oil (1 tablespoon)

- Minced garlic (1 teaspoon)

- Ripe tomatoes–chopped (.5 cup)

- Drained capers (1 tablespoon)

- Zucchini noodles (4 cups)

- Salt and black pepper (as desired)

- Fresh parsley–chopped (1 tablespoon)

- Optional: Parmesan cheese

Directions:

1.   Open the can of sardines. Pour the oil into a large sauté pan using the med-high temperature setting. Mix the olive oil and the sardine oil.

2.   Chop and toss in the garlic. Sauté for one minute or until fragrant and sizzling.

3.   Drain and add the capers and tomatoes. Simmer for one minute.

4.   Mix in the sardines and simmer for another minute.

5.   Mix in the zucchini noodles and gently stir so you don't break up the sardines too much. Simmer for two minutes – or longer if you like them soft.

6.   Garnish with parsley, salt, and pepper. Serve hot with a dusting of parmesan cheese.

Nutrition: Calories: 324 Fat,: 16 g Carb1 2 g Protein: 13 g

Spicy Korean Beef Noodles

Preparation time: 10 minutes

Cooking time: 15 minutes

Serves: 4

Ingredients:

- 1/2 tablespoon extra-virgin olive oil

- 1/2 red onion, sliced thin

- 1 garlic clove, minced

- 1 pound flank steak, sliced thin

- 1 small to medium cabbage, spiralized (napa cabbage would be good for this)

- 1 to 2 teaspoons chili garlic oil or chili garlic sauce

- 11/2 tablespoons sesame oil

- 1 tablespoon coconut aminos

- 1/2 large cucumber, diced, for garnish

- 2 or 3 green onions, chopped, for garnish

- 2 to 3 tablespoons chopped fresh cilantro, for garnish

Directions:

1. In a large skillet over medium heat, heat the olive oil and sauté the red onion for about 5 minutes. Add the garlic

and the steak and cook the steak pieces for about 3 minutes per side.

2.   Add the cabbage to the skillet and sauté for 3 to 4 minutes, or until the cabbage noodles are beginning to wilt. Lower the heat to medium-low and add the chili garlic oil, sesame oil, and coconut aminos. Stir until combined and remove from the heat.

3.   Spoon into bowls, garnish with the cucumber, green onions, and cilantro, and serve.

Nutrition: Calories 112 Fat 9g, Protein 2g, Carbs 5g, Fiber 2g

Keto Butter Cabbage Noodles

Preparation time: 5 minutes

Cooking time: 10 minutes

Servings: 2

Ingredients:

- A quarter cup of unsalted butter

- A teaspoon of dried oregano

- A clove of garlic (diced)

- Half a cup of parmesan cheese (shredded)

- A teaspoon of salt

- A teaspoon of dried basil

- A head of green cabbage

- A quarter cup of red pepper flakes

- Half a bulb of onion

Directions:

1.   Wash the cabbage and cut into thin long strips then set aside.

2.   Dice the onion and garlic then set aside

3.   Melt butter on medium -high in a non-stick frying pan

4.   Saute the minced onion and garlic until they start to brown.

5.   Add chili flakes, salt and herbs and stir until well combined.

6.   Add the cabbage and stir until it is fully coated in the mixture.

7.   Cook for 2-3 minutes or until it loses moisture and starts to wilt.

8.   Note: If you cook it for too long, it will lose too much moisture and become too soft. We want it to have a spaghetti feel to it, so turn it down when it can perfectly fold around a fork.

9.   Put the cabbage in a plate and sprinkle some parmesan cheese on top then serve.

10.   You can spice up your cabbage noodles with some diced chicken, bacon or minced beef.

Nutrition: Calories: 187 Total Fat: 5g Carbs: 1g Protein: 3g

KETO CHAFFLE

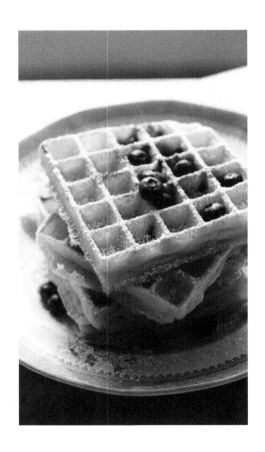

Quinoa Parmigiano-Reggiano Chaffles

Preparation Time: 5 minutes

Cooking Time: 5 minutes

Servings: 2

Ingredients:

• Parmigiano-Reggiano cheese (shredded) – 1 cup

• Eggs – 2

• Quinoa flour – 2 tablespoons

Directions:

1. Pre-heat and grease waffle iron

2. Mix Parmigiano-Reggiano cheese and eggs in one bowl

3. Add the Quinoa flour into mixture to enhance texture

4. Pour mixture onto waffle plate and cook till crunchy

5. Garnish ready and slightly cooled chaffles with preferred garnish

6. Takes 5 min to prepare and serves 2

Nutrition: Calories 115 Fat 7.3g Protein 1.4g Carbs: 4g

Bacon and Sour Cream Chaffles

Preparation Time: 5 minutes

Cooking Time: 20 minutes

Servings: 2

Ingredients:

- Cheddar – 1 cup

- Sour cream – 3 tablespoons

- American cheese – 2 slices

- Bacon pieces – 4

- Sour cream – 2 tablespoons

Directions:

1. Pre-heat and grease waffle maker

2. Mix Sour cream and cheddar cheese together

3. Pour mixture onto waffle plate and cook till crunchy

4. Cook bacon pieces till crispy then dry then

5. Fry Sour cream and add it in between two chaffles alongside bacon and cheese slices

Nutrition: Calories 115 Fat 7.3g Protein 1.4g Carbs: 4g

Zucchini Bel Paese Chaffles

Preparation Time: 12 minutes

Cooking Time: 30 minutes

Servings: 4

Ingredients:

• 	Grated zucchini – 1

• 	Eggs – 1

• 	Shredded Bel Paese – 1/2 cup

• 	Parmesan – 1 tablespoon

• 	Pepper (as desired)

• 	Oregano – 1 teaspoon

Directions:

1. 	Pre-heat waffle iron

2. 	Add all ingredients in one bowl then mix thoroughly

3. 	Grease waffle iron and pour mixture into waffle plate

4. 	Cook till crispy

Nutrition: Calories 76 Total Fat 7.2 g Total Carbs 2g Sugar 1 g

Fiber 0.7 g Protein 2.2 g

Crispy American Grana Chaffles

Preparation Time: 12 minutes

Cooking Time: 30 minutes

Servings: 4

Ingredients:

- Cheddar cheese (shredded) – 1/3 cup
- Eggs – 1
- Baking powder – 1/4 teaspoon
- Chia seeds (ground) – 1 teaspoon
- American Grana cheese (shredded) – 1/3 cup

Directions:

1.   Mix all ingredients except American Grana cheese in one bowl

2.   Shred half American Grana cheese on waffle iron to grease plate

3.   Pour mixture and top with remaining shredded American Grana cheese

4.   Cook till crispy

Nutrition: Calories: 125 Fat: 7g Carb: 1 g Protein: 5g

Shiitake Chaffles

Preparation Time: 4 minutes

Cooking Time: 10 minutes

Servings: 4

Ingredients:

- Caciocavallo – 1/2 cup

- Eggs – 2

- Baking powder – 1/2 teaspoon

- Asparagus (finely cut) – 1/4 cup

- For Toppings

- Shiitake mushrooms – 4 tablespoons

- Kewpie mayonnaise – 2 tablespoons

- Seaweed powder – 2 tablespoons

- Beni shoga – 2 tablespoons

- Green onion stalk– 1

- For sauce

- Soy sauce – 4 teaspoons

- Ketchup – 4 tablespoons

- Worcestershire/Worcester sauce – 4 teaspoons

- Stevia sweetener – 2 tablespoons

Directions:

1.   Mix sauce ingredients in a separate bowl

2.   Pre-heat waffle maker and grease

3.   Beat eggs in separate bowl

4.   Add finely cut asparagus, baking powder and Caciocavallo cheese then mix

5.   Pour mixture onto waffle plate and cook till crisp

6.   Top chaffles with seaweed powder , bonito flakes, chopped onions and Beni Shoga

7.   Spread kewpie sauce and okonomiyaki sauce

Nutrition: Calories 195 Total Fat 14.3 g Total Carbs 4.5 g Sugar 0.5 g Fiber 0.3 g Protein 3.2 g

Cheese Curds Chaffles

Preparation Time: 4 minutes

Cooking Time: 10 minutes

Servings: 4

Ingredients:

• Ketchup – 2 tablespoons

• Cheese Curds – 3 oz

Directions:

1. Cut Cheese Curds cheese into half inch slices

2. Place cheese in waffle maker then turn on

3. Cook for about 6 min till golden brown

4. Spread sauce on chaffle

5. Takes 5 min to prepare and 6 min to cook and serves 2 – serve hot.

Nutrition: Calories 252 Total Fat 17.3 g Total Carbs 3.2 g Sugar 0.3 g Fiber 1.4 g Protein 5.2 g

MAIN, SIDE & VEGETABLE

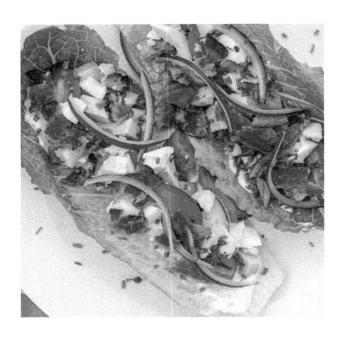

Cheesy Garlic Salmon

Preparation time: 15 minutes

Cooking time: 12 minutes

Servings:4

Ingredients:

- ½ cup Asiago cheese
- 2 tablespoons freshly squeezed lemon juice
- 2 tablespoons butter, at room temperature
- 2 teaspoons minced garlic
- teaspoon chopped fresh basil
- teaspoon chopped fresh oregano
- 4 (5-ounce) salmon fillets
- tablespoon olive oil

Directions:

1.   Preheat the oven to 350°F. Line a baking sheet with parchment paper and set aside.

2.   In a small bowl, stir together the Asiago cheese, lemon juice, butter, garlic, basil, and oregano.

3.   Pat the salmon dry with paper towels and place the fillets on the baking sheet skin-side down. Divide the topping evenly between the fillets and spread it across the fish using a knife or the back of a spoon.

4.   Drizzle the fish with the olive oil and bake until the topping is golden and the fish is just cooked through, about 12 minutes.

5.   Serve.

Nutrition: Calories: 357 Fat: 28g Protein: 24g Carbohydrates: 2g Fiber: 0g

Broccoli and Mozzarella Muffins

Preparation time: 5 minutes

Cooking time: 12 minutes

Servings: 2

Ingredients:

- 1/3 cup chopped broccoli
- 2 eggs
- tbsp coconut cream
- tbsp grated mozzarella cheese, full-fat
- Seasoning:
- ¼ tsp salt
- ¼ tsp ground black pepper

Directions:

1. Turn on the oven, then set it to 350 degrees F and let it preheat.

2. Take a medium bowl, crack eggs in it and whisk in salt, black pepper, and cream until well combined.

3. Add broccoli and cheese, stir until mixed, divide the batter evenly between two silicone muffin cups, and bake for 10 to 12 minutes until firm and the top has golden brown.

4.	When done, let muffin cool for 5 minutes, then take them out and serve.

Nutrition: 135 Calories; 9.5 g Fats; 9.1 g Protein; 1.4 g Net Carb; 0.6 g Fiber;

Sole Asiago

Preparation time: 10 minutes

Cooking time: 8 minutes

Servings: 4

Ingredients:

•   4 (4-ounce) sole fillets

•   ¾ cup ground almonds

•   ¼ cup Asiago cheese

•   2 eggs, beaten

•   2½ tablespoons melted coconut oil

Directions:

1.   Preheat the oven to 350°F. Line a baking sheet with parchment paper and set aside.

2.   Pat the fish dry with paper towels.

3.   Stir together the ground almonds and cheese in a small bowl.

4.   Place the bowl with the beaten eggs in it next to the almond mixture.

5. Dredge a sole fillet in the beaten egg and then press the fish into the almond mixture so it is completely coated. Place on the baking sheet and repeat until all the fillets are breaded.

6. Brush both sides of each piece of fish with the coconut oil.

7. Bake the sole until it is cooked through, about 8 minutes in total.

8. Serve immediately.

Nutrition: Calories: 406 Fat: 31g Protein: 29g carbohydrates: 6g Fiber: 3g

Buttered Broccoli

Preparation Time: 10 minutes

Cooking Time: 15 minutes

Servings: 4

Ingredients:

- 2 medium heads broccoli, cut into florets
- 2 garlic cloves, minced
- ¼ C. butter, melted
- 2 tbsp. fresh lemon juice
- tsp. Italian seasoning
- Salt and freshly ground black pepper, to taste

Directions:

1. Preheat the oven to 450 degrees F.
2. In a bowl, add all ingredients and toss to coat well.
3. Place broccoli mixture into a large baking dish and spread in a single layer.
4. Bake for about 12-15 minutes.
5. Serve hot.

Nutrition: Calories 109; Carbohydrates: 7.4g; Protein: 3.1g; Fat: 12.3g; Sugar: 2g; Sodium: 155mg; Fiber: 2.6g

Zucchini Breakfast Hash

Preparation time: 5 minutes

Cooking time: 15 minutes

Servings: 2

Ingredients:

- 4 slices of bacon, chopped

- zucchini, diced

- eggs

- tbsp avocado oil

- Seasoning:

- 3/4 tsp salt, divided

- ¼ tsp ground black pepper

Directions:

1. Take a skillet pan, place it over medium heat, add bacon, and cook for 5 minutes until lightly brown.

2. Then add zucchini, season with ½ tsp salt, stir, cook for 10 minutes and then transfer to plate.

3.   Fry eggs to desired level in avocado oil, season eggs with salt and black pepper to taste and serve with zucchini hash.

Nutrition: 144.5 Calories; 12.5 g Fats; 6 g Protein; 0.9 g Net Carb; 0.5 g Fiber;

Great Side Dish

Preparation Time: 10 minutes

Cooking Time: 15 minutes

Servings: 3

Ingredients:

- 2 C. broccoli florets

- small yellow onion, cut into wedges

- ½ tsp. garlic powder

- 1/8 tsp. paprika

- Freshly ground black pepper, to taste

- tbsp. butter, melted

Directions:

1. Preheat the grill to medium heat.

2. In a large bowl, add all ingredients and toss to coat well.

3. Transfer the broccoli mixture over a double thickness of a foil paper.

4. Fold the foil around broccoli mixture to seal it.

5. Grill for about 10-15 minutes.

6. Serve hot.

Nutrition: Calories 99; Carbohydrates: 6.5g; Protein: 2.1g; Fat: 7.9g; Sugar: 2.1g; Sodium: 76mg; Fiber: 2.1g

Bacon, Avocado Egg Boats

Preparation time: 5 minutes

Cooking time: 15 minutes

Servings: 2

Ingredients:

- avocado, pitted
- slices of turkey bacon
- eggs
- Seasoning:
- ¼ tsp salt
- 1/8 tsp ground black pepper

Directions:

1.	Turn on the oven, then set it to 425 degrees F and let it preheat.

2.	Meanwhile, prepare the avocado and for this, cut the avocado into half, remove the pit and then scoop out some of the flesh to make the hollow bigger.

3.   Take a skillet pan, place it over medium heat and when hot, add bacon slices and cook for 3 minutes per side until crisp.

4.   Transfer each slice into the hollow of each avocado half, crack the egg into each hollow and bake the egg boats for 12 to 15 minutes until the egg has cooked to the desired level.

5.   When done, season egg boats with salt and black pepper and serve.

Nutrition: 229 Calories; 18 g Fats; 11 g Protein; 1.1 g Net Carb; 4.6 g Fiber;

SOUP AND STEWS

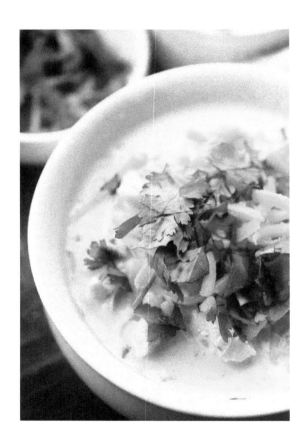

Italian Beef Soup

Preparation time: 10 minutes

Cooking time: 4 hours

Servings:6

Ingredients:

- pound lean ground beef

- cup beef broth

- cup heavy cream

- ½ cup shredded mozzarella cheese

- ½ cup diced tomatoes

- 1 yellow onion, chopped

- cloves garlic, chopped

- 1 tablespoon Italian seasoning

- Salt & pepper, to taste

Directions:

1. Add all the ingredients to a slow cooker minus the heavy cream and mozzarella cheese. Cook on high for 4 hours.

2. Warm the heavy cream, and then add the warmed cream and cheese to the soup. Stir well and serve.

Nutrition: Calories: 241 Carbs: 4g Fiber: 1g Net Carbs: 3g Fat: 14g Protein: 25g

Pumpkin, Coconut & Sage Soup

Preparation time: 15 minutes

Cooking time: 30 minutes

Servings:6

Ingredients:

- 6 cups vegetable broth

- cup canned pumpkin

- cup full-fat coconut milk

- teaspoon freshly chopped sage

- cloves garlic, chopped

- Pinch of salt & pepper, to taste

Directions:

1.   Add all the ingredients minus the coconut milk to a stockpot over medium heat and bring to a boil. Reduce to a simmer and cook for 30 minutes.

2.   Add the coconut milk and stir.

Nutrition: Calories: 146 Carbs: 7g Fiber: 2g Net Carbs: 5g Fat: 11g Protein: 6g

Chili Cheese Taco Dip

Preparation Time: 10 minutes

Cooking Time: 45 minutes

Servings: 16

Ingredients:

- 1-pound ground beef

- 1-pound mild Mexican cheese, grated

- can tomato salsa

- packet Mexican spice blend

- can tomato sauce

- Salt and pepper to taste

- 1 cup water

Directions:

1.   Heat a heavy-bottomed pot on medium heat and sauté the ground beef until browned, around 10 minutes. Season with pepper and salt.

2.   Add tomato salsa, Mexican spice blend, and tomato sauce. Bring to a boil, lower fire to a simmer, and simmer for 25 minutes.

3.   Stir in half of the cheese and mix well. Continue simmering until well-combined, around 10 minutes more.

4.   Sprinkle remaining cheese on top and serve.

Nutrition: Calories: 160 Fat: 11.3g Carbs: 1.6g Protein: 12.4g

DESSERT

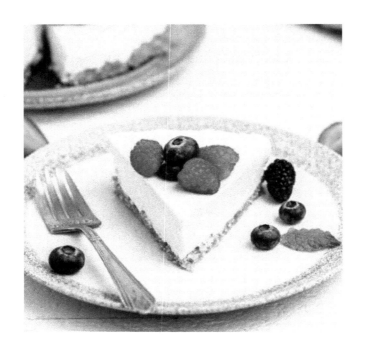

Pumpkin Cheesecake Cookies

Preparation Time: 10 minutes

Cooking Time: 20 minutes

Servings: 12

Ingredients:

- For the Pumpkin Cookie

- 6 tbsp. butter, softened

- 2 cups almond flour

- 1/3 cup solid pack pumpkin puree

- 1 large egg

- 3/4 cup granulated erythritol sweetener

- 1/2 tsp. baking powder

- 1 tsp. ground cinnamon

- 1/4 tsp. ground nutmeg

- 1/8 tsp. ground allspice

- Pinch of salt

- For the Cheesecake Filling

- 4 oz. cream cheese

- 1/2 tsp. vanilla

- 1 large egg

- 2 tbsp. granulated erythritol sweetener

Directions:

1. Preheat your oven at 350 degrees F.

2. Add all the cookie dough ingredients to a suitable bowl and form a smooth dough.

3. Add the dough to a cookie sheet lined with wax paper scoop by scoop.

4. Flatten the scoops of dough with a spoon and make a dent in the center of each cookie.

5. Whisk cream cheese with vanilla, egg, and sweetener in a mixer.

6. Divide this mixture into the center of each cookie.

7. Bake them for 20 minutes until golden brown.

8. Allow them to cool for 10 minutes.

9. Enjoy.

Nutrition: Calories 175 Total Fat 16 G Total Carbs 2.8 G Sugar 1.8 G Fiber 0.4 G Protein 9 G

Pecan Shortbread Cookies

Preparation Time: 5 minutes

Cooking Time: 15 minutes

Servings: 6

Ingredients:

- 3/4 cup almond flour

- 1/4 cup coconut flour

- 1 large egg

- 4 tbsp butter, melted

- 1/2 cup erythritol

- 1 tsp vanilla extract

- 1/2 tsp baking powder

- 1/4 tsp xanthan gum

- 1/3 cup raw pecans, crushed

Directions:

1. Add all dry ingredients to a bowl then mix well with a fork.

2. Whisk melted butter and vanilla extract in a separate bowl then stir in half of the dry mixture.

3. Add egg and mix well until combined. Now, stir in the remaining dry mixture.

4. Mix this well until fully incorporated.

5. Add pecans to the cookie dough and mix well.

6. Place the dough on wax paper and form it into a rectangular log with your hands.

7. Cover it with more wax paper and freeze for 30 minutes.

8. Meanwhile, preheat your oven for 5 minutes at 350 degrees F.

9. Layer a cookie sheet with wax paper and set it aside.

10. Slice the dough log into 1/4-inch thick slices.

11. Place the slices on the cookie sheet and bake them for 15 minutes.

12. Allow them to cool then serve.

Nutrition: Calories 121 Total Fat 12.9 g Carbs 2.1 g Sugar 1.8 g Fiber 0.4 g Protein 5.4 g

Cinnamon Roll Muffins

Preparation Time: 5 minutes

Cooking Time: 15 minutes

Servings: 6

Ingredients:

- 1/2 cup almond flour

- 2 scoops vanilla protein powder

- 1 tsp. baking powder

- 1 tbsp. cinnamon

- 1/2 cup almond butter

- 1/2 cup pumpkin puree

- 1/2 cup coconut oil

- For the Glaze

- 1/4 cup coconut butter

- 1/4 cup milk of choice

- 1 tbsp. granulated sweetener

- 2 tsp. lemon juice

Directions:

1.   Let your oven preheat at 350 degrees F. Layer a 12-cup muffin tray with muffin liners.

2. Add all the dry ingredients to a suitable mixing bowl then whisk in all the wet ingredients.

3. Mix until well combined then divide the batter into the muffin cups.

4. Bake them for 15 minutes then allow the muffins to cool on a wire rack.

5. Prepare the cinnamon glaze in a small bowl then drizzle this glaze over the muffins.

6. Enjoy.

Nutrition: Calories 252 Total Fat 17.3 g Total Carbs 3.2 g Sugar 0.3 g Fiber 1.4 g Protein 5.2 g

Muffins with Blueberries

Preparation Time: 10 minutes

Cooking Time: 25 minutes

Servings: 8

Ingredients:

- 3/4 cup coconut flour

- 6 eggs

- 1/2 cup coconut oil, melted

- 1/3 cup unsweetened coconut milk

- 1/2 cup fresh blueberries

- 1/3 cup granulated sweetener

- 1 tsp. vanilla extract

- 1 tsp. baking powder

Directions:

1. Preheat your oven at 356 degrees F.

2. Mix coconut flour with all the other ingredients except blueberries in a mixing bowl until smooth.

3. Stir in blueberries and mix gently.

4. Divide this batter in a greased muffin tray evenly.

5. Bake the muffins for 25 minutes until golden brown.

6.   Enjoy.

Nutrition: Calories 195 Total Fat 14.3 g Total Carbs 4.5 g Sugar 0.5 g Fiber 0.3 g Protein 3.2 g

Keto Thumbprint Cookies

Preparation Time: 10 minutes

Cooking Time: 8 minutes

Servings: 8

Ingredients:

- 1 large egg, beaten

- 1/2 cup salted butter, softened

- 2 cups superfine blanched almond flour

- Pinch of kosher salt

- 1/2 tsp. baking powder

- 2/3 cup powdered erythritol sweetener

- 1 tsp. vanilla extract

- 1/3 cup finely chopped walnuts

- 5 tbsp. sugar-free strawberry preserves

Directions:

1.   Preheat your oven to 375 degrees F.

2.   Beat egg with almond flour, vanilla, butter, salt, erythritol, baking powder, and vanilla in a medium bowl.

3.   Make 1.5-inch balls out of this mixture and flatten them slightly.

4.   Top these cookies with the walnuts then place them on a baking sheet lined with wax paper.

5.   Bake them for 8 minutes then make small grooves in the center of each cookie.

6.   Add a teaspoon of jam into the center of each cookie then bake them for 10 minutes.

7.   Let them cool down completely.

8.   Serve.

Nutrition: Calories 190 Total Fat 17.5 g Total Carbs 2.5 g Sugar 2.8 g Fiber 3.8 g Protein 3 g

Keto Chocolate Chip Cookies

Preparation Time: 10 minutes

Cooking Time: 16 minutes

Servings: 8

Ingredients:

•   1 cup sunflower seed butter

•   2 eggs

•   1/4 cup coconut flour

•   1 tsp. vanilla extract

•   1 cup granulated erythritol sweetener

•   1/4 cup unsweetened shredded coconut

•   1 tbsp. konjac flour

•   1/4 tsp. kosher salt

•   2 oz. coarsely chopped Lindt 90% dark chocolate

Directions:

1.   Preheat your oven to 350 degrees F.

2.   Mix sunflower seed butter with vanilla, coconut flour, eggs, sweetener, shredded coconut, salt, and konjac flour in a suitably sized bowl.

3.   Mix well then fold in chopped chocolate.

4.   Make 15 balls out of this mixture then place them on a baking sheet lined with wax paper.

5.   Gently press the balls to flatten them into cookies.

6.   Bake these cookies for 16 minutes until golden brown.

7.   Allow them to cool then garnish with salt flakes.

8.   Enjoy.

Nutrition: Calories 285 Total Fat 17.3 g Total Carbs 3.5 g Sugar 0.4 g Fiber 0.9 g Protein 7.2 g

Lightning Source UK Ltd.
Milton Keynes UK
UKHW020714270521
384463UK00001B/35